Hepatitis C

Symptoms,

Treatment

and Cure

Hepatitis C Symptoms, Treatment and Cure

Dennis Clause

Disclaimer

This book is dedicated to
Laura Harding N.P.

Thank you

Contents

This is not an advice book!

Seek a doctor for any medical advice!

Chapter 1
Hepatitis C Symptoms

Most people don't know that there are symptoms of Hepatitis C that go undiagnosed for many years because it rarely causes symptoms in its early stage. Actually, someone who has been carrying Hepatitis C for decades may not have any symptoms until it has caused a significant liver damage. Even then, the symptoms typically appear and disappear.

When indicators of liver disease finally surface, they can range from mild to severe. The most common symptom of which is the universal vague problem of tiredness.

Another common symptom of Hepatitis C includes irregular stomach discomfort. The liver is on the right side of the mid-section, just under the rib cage. When the liver is infected, it can cause pain or discomfort, however, some people don't actually experience pain but they do feel a broad sense of fullness.

Abdominal pain from Hepatitis C is not always within the liver region. It can also be described to be coming from other areas of the mid-section.

Since the liver is an integral part of the body's gastrointestinal system, Hepatitis C can cause: Reduced appetite, weight loss, nausea, or vomiting. Depression also generally accompanies Hepatitis C infection.

Specialists have proposed a range of factors revealing why those with Hepatitis C get depressed. Whereas there is no single, mutually agreed upon reason, there isn't any doubt that depression is very common in people with Hepatitis C infection.

Jaundice usually does not appear in the early stage of Hepatitis C infection, however, this condition of the skin or whites of the eyes is a sure sign of advancing liver disease.

Another measure of advancing liver disease can be seen in the form of dark-colored urine and light- or grey-colored stool. If Hepatitis C has already caused a permanent scarring of the liver, known as Cirrhosis, the following symptoms may be a sign of this complication.

Fluid retention may cause swelling of the stomach (also known as ascites) and puffiness in the legs or the whole body.

Skin itching is typical when the liver is unable to filter the blood of toxins. Bleeding (eg, coughing up blood or vomiting of blood) results from an extremely high level of strain in the liver.

Confusion, hallucinations, or extreme sleepiness may be the consequences of toxins accumulating in the blood and affecting the brain. Because Cirrhosis and its complications (mostly vomiting of blood or confusion) can be dangerous, they must be treated instantly.

Even though the symptoms mentioned previously are the most commonly experienced indicators of Hepatitis C, they're certainly not exclusive.

In recent times, medical specialists have learned to admit extra hepatic symptoms of Hepatitis C, where issues arise outside of the liver. Additionally, patients undergoing medical treatment for Hepatitis C are more likely susceptible to the medication's side effects which can be quite unpleasant.

As you can tell, the symptoms connected with Hepatitis C are indistinct, and infrequently prompt people to visit a physician. As a matter of fact, approximately 80% of those newly infected with the virus won't have any symptoms at all. Unfortunately, when someone with Hepatitis C see a doctor due to severe symptoms, usually the disease has already progressed to advanced liver disease.

Since a lot of people may live with this virus for 10 or 20 years without symptoms, anyone who has risk factors or suspecting they have the virus should call for a Hepatitis C test. That way, if they test positive, they can consider the treatment against Hepatitis C and prevent further harm to their liver.

Hepatitis C affects countless Americans, yet it continues to be one of the most poorly understood diseases.

Chapter 2
10 Basic Misconceptions

#1, If I have Hepatitis C, it would have interfered with my health and I would probably have the symptoms. Hepatitis C is usually labeled as a silent killer because it can be an asymptomatic disease. Between 80% and 85% of those with Hepatitis C have no signs or symptoms of their infection, and they may not surface until it is too late.

#2, Hepatitis C is a death sentence. Even though this illness may be dormant for a long time, it can be treated. If you feel unwell for no particular reason, see a doctor and have yourself checked up. Have your blood tested if you ever had blood transfusion, had injected needles, have HIV or born to a mother with Hepatitis C.#3, Hepatitis C viral load correlates with disease progression. Though it is realistic to assume that a higher viral load indicates that Hepatitis C has progressed more rapidly, investigation does not verify this. There is no correlation between the number of virus in a person's blood and their level of liver damage. Laboratory tests and a liver biopsy are just some of the ways to determine the extent of liver damage. Even though Hepatitis C is so prevalent, there is still a lack of understanding regarding this virus. By learning more about Hepatitis C, and being able to distinguish between a fact and a myth, our society will have a better idea of what this illness is about, how to handle it, and how they can protect themselves from this contagious disease.

#4 You can get Hepatitis C from taking an excessive amount of alcohol. This is definitely not true. Hepatitis C is caused by a virus, however, consuming alcohol will worsen Hepatitis C infection. There are different kinds of hepatitis and hepatitis caused by excessive intake of alcohol is known as Alcoholic Hepatitis.

#5, Hepatitis C medical treatment is always difficult. Although the treatment for Hepatitis C consists of combinations of drugs which may cause unpleasant or severe side effects, there are plenty of individuals who completed their treatment regimen with no problem. In addition, patients who followed a healthy lifestyle seemed to complete the Hepatitis C treatment easier.

#6, If you have received a vaccination for hepatitis, you don't need to bother about Hepatitis C. Unfortunately, there is no vaccine for Hepatitis C yet. Vaccines for Hepatitis A and Hepatitis B are available, but they don't offer protection against Hepatitis C.

#7, A man on Hepatitis C combination therapy does not need to worry about getting a woman pregnant. Certain medications cause birth defects and may cause fetal loss, hence men taking Interferon and Ribavirin are strictly advised to use 2 forms of contraception throughout treatment, and for 6 months following treatment.

#8, Hepatitis C is a sexually transmitted disease. It is possible to transmit Hepatitis C through sexual contact only if you come into contact with contaminated blood of the infected person during intercourse which does not happen very often. Since merely a minimal percentage of Hepatitis C is believed to be contracted through sex, Hepatitis C is not considered a sexually transmitted disease.

#9, HIV, the virus that causes AIDS, is more prevalent and contagious than Hepatitis C. Although the public knows more facts about HIV than Hepatitis C, Hepatitis C displays larger health hazard because it infects over 4 times more Americans, and is 7 times more spreadable than HIV.

#10, Those with Hepatitis C are drug users. Intravenous drug use may be the simplest route of Hepatitis C infection but there are many other ways to transmit this blood-borne virus. In fact, up to a third of people infected with Hepatitis C are unable to identify the source of their infection.

Chapter 3
Some Facts

Now, I want to write about the sexual transmission of the Hepatitis C virus. Approximately 4 million Americans are presumed to be a carrier of Hepatitis C. As the number of individuals becoming aware that they have this spreadable disease is continuing to rise, so is the concern of how they were initially infected with this disease. Medical experts agree that Hepatitis C is primarily transmitted through blood. While the majority of Hepatitis C infections are contracted through intravenous drug use or tainted blood transfusions, an estimated 10-30% of those infected, have no idea how they got Hepatitis C in the first place.

With such a significant number of people infected with this virus who are unclear about how their disease was obtained, just about every opportunity become believable. Medical specialists are not consistent about the sexual transmission of Hepatitis C. While some assure their patients that getting Hepatitis C from sex is rare, others tell those infected that they probably got it from sexual intercourse.

When someone learns he/she has Hepatitis C, there is often a great fear of passing the virus to his/her partner. In general, the science has concluded a remarkably low occurrence of transmitting Hepatitis C through sexual contact. For people infected with Hepatitis C who are in a monogamous relationship, the risk of sexual transmission ranges from 0-0.6% per year. This risk of transmission is moderately higher, about 1% per year, for those who are involved in short-term sexual relationships. This risk rises if the infected partner is co-infected with HIV.

Some studies, specifically considering monogamous, heterosexual relationships, found that the probability of sexually transmitting Hepatitis C is either low or non-existent. According to the Hepatitis C partner study completed by the Center for Disease Control in 2004, the risk of sexual transmission in the United States is 2.2% in monogamous, heterosexual relationships where one partner has Hepatitis C.

As published in May 2004 edition of The American Journal of Gastroenterology, investigators found that the risk of sexual transmission of Hepatitis C within heterosexual, monogamous couples is incredibly low, or perhaps null. As published in April 2005 edition of The American Journal of Gastroenterology, researchers found that out of 216 Hepatitis C-negative individuals who had sexual intercourse with Hepatitis C-positive partners of the opposite sex, zero obtained Hepatitis C during their 3-year period study.

While the risk of transmitting Hepatitis C in heterosexual, monogamous couples is incredibly low, there are a number of factors that increase risk of transmission. The risk increases in the following 4 situations.

The first is HIV. When the individual infected with Hepatitis C is also infected with HIV, there is a much higher risk of passing Hepatitis C. Although scientists don't yet understand why, it seems that those who are co-infected have greater quantities of Hepatitis C genetic material in both seminal and vaginal fluids.

The 2nd is high viral load. When someone with Hepatitis C has a high viral load, the probability of passing the virus increases.

The third is having different partners.

Several studies have demonstrated that those who have frequent encounters with multiple sexual partners have a high risk of contracting Hepatitis C.

The fourth is hard sex. Since the membranes that line our sexual organs are more fragile than other parts of the body, they are more vulnerable to injury.

When this mucosa is injured from vigorous sexual techniques such as anal intercourse, fisting, and the use of certain sex toys, the risk of bleeding increases, and thus the risk of Hepatitis C transmission also increases.

The risk of transmitting Hepatitis C through sexual contact is low, especially for heterosexual, monogamous partners who do not have the risk factors formerly described. However, there is enough evidence that sexual transmission of Hepatitis C is possible, mostly because many infected patients do not know how they contracted it to begin with.

Until definite guidelines are established on how to prevent the spread of this virus, practicing safe sex is the only trustworthy solution to prevent the sexual transmission of Hepatitis C.

Chapter 4
Good and Bad Foods

Better heath starts with eating the right kinds of food. Most people recognize the value of food in addressing health issues. Since everything we eat is processed by the liver, people with any form of liver disease should be extra careful on the kind of food they eat. Because chronic Hepatitis C locks the liver in a constant battle against inflammation, food choices are significant to people managing this virus. Unfortunately, dietary advice quite often gets lost in the shuffle of dealing with Hepatitis C control and treatment. To make matters even worse, some insurance companies don't cover nutritionists, despite the massive contribution these professionals do to people with chronic liver disease.

Because certain foods can cause inflammation in the liver, eating an unsuitable food can intensify liver damage and worsen the condition of a person with Hepatitis C.

To avoid this, steer clear of consuming items in the following 5 categories.

The first product to abstain from is alcohol. Right from the start of Hepatitis C diagnosis, complete alcohol abstinence is non-negotiated. Technically, most of us don't consider alcohol as food, but drinking is the most obvious way to introduce poisonous substances to the liver. Like throwing gasoline on a fire, alcohol will exponentially increase Hepatitis C viral load.

The second category to avoid, or at least minimize, is fast food. While most people will possibly not think their lunch is toxic, millions of Americans damage their liver by eating fast food. Even a brief fast food binge combined with too little exercise can cause liver damage. When we overload the liver with extreme calories and fat, its ability to filter the blood leads to fat and toxins buildup and consequently result to liver damage. Thus, the lure of a quick burger and fries is extremely dangerous to those with Hepatitis C.

The third food group to restrict is high glycemic index car-

bohydrates. By measuring how quickly foods are digested and absorbed, the glycemic index measures the body's response to carbohydrates. Carbohydrates with a high glycemic index are absorbed quickly into the blood stream, and cause a rapid rise in blood glucose levels. Research shows a direct relationship between carbohydrates with a high glycemic index and fatty liver.

Unfortunately, fat buildup in the liver accelerates the damage done by the Hepatitis C virus. Some popular, high glycemic index foods to restrict are: Potatoes, corn, white flour, white rice, refined sugar, and refined breakfast cereals.

The fourth dietary rule is to minimize iron-rich foods. While this category only involves foods with high iron levels, approximately 30% of people with Hepatitis C are affected. Because excessive iron in the liver worsens the progression of Hepatitis C, individuals who have elevated iron counts must limit their iron intake. This means eating little amounts of red meat, ensuring that vitamins being taken do not contain iron, not using cast iron cookware, and making sure not to take vitamin C supplementations and consume plant sources of iron such as spinach or beets at the same time because vitamin C enhances iron's absorption. The fifth nutrition rule for people infected with Hepatitis C is to avoid dirty produce. Because most economically grown produce is slathered with poisonous pesticides, unwashed produce puts an additional toxic burden on the liver. To prevent the additional damage that these toxins do to a liver battling Hepatitis C, make sure to completely wash commercially grown fruits and veggies.

Because seeing a nutritionist may not be within everyone's grasp, avoiding alcohol, fast food, high glycemic index carbohydrates, foods high in iron, and unwashed produce will in place of a personalized, professionally crafted eating plan benefit people with Hepatitis C.

Chapter 5

My Story

Hello, now this is the part of my story where I talk about uh finding out I had Hepatitis C.

When I decided to quit drugs, I was able to put the drugs down but I had problem quitting alcohol. So I moved to Tennessee and stayed with some family members, cousins and aunt to help me get on my feet. While I was there, I planned to go to a rehab but decided to see a doctor first to get checked out for anything just so I would know for my own sake which is um you know HIV, STDs, anything like that. And so I got the blood work done. When the result of the blood tests came, the doctor explained that I don't have HIV nor STDs, but I do have Hepatitis C. And I remember looking at her as she tells me that I have Hepatitis C,

I couldn't understand any word that she was saying after that. It was funny because I'm looking at her and I know she was talking but it wasn't processing in my brain. The only thing I could think of was, "Oh my goodness I can't believe this is happening to me. This is not supposed to happen to me, this doesn't happen to people like me. I'm a decent person, I didn't share needles, I didn't have unprotected sex, I didn't do any of that. How could this possibly happen to me?"

As as she was talking, I asked her, "could you start all over again? I didn't understand any of what you said," and so she did. But again, I didn't understand a word that the doctor was saying. I just looked at her and said, "Can I have a few minutes to process this? I do not fully believe this… I don't uh.. it, it's not clicking." She said, "Okay, I'll go see my next patient to give you some time to think about it. I'll be back." She also said, "Right there on the wall, is a pamphlet about Hepatitis C" before leaving. As I was reading the pamphlet, I think to myself, "I can't believe this happened, this is not the plan, this isn't true, maybe she can test it again because uh she's wrong, the doctor's wrong."When the doctor came back after ten or fifteen minutes, she started explaining about Hepatitis C, what to look out for, and that there should be no alcohol, no aspirin, and everything that is bad for the liver. The doctor was a very nice person and was very patient with me. I said, "Well, is there a cure?" And the doctor said, "There's no cure." And I took it as, "The doctor didn't lie to me, the doctor didn't know, a lot of people don't know that there is a possible cure, treatment, so the doctor didn't lie to me, the doctor just didn't know."

So I took the doctor's word as, "That's it then; that's all." So I got some pamphlets and other information and I uh went back to the house I was staying at. I couldn't decide if I will tell anybody, or keep it a secret, or what should I do.

Chapter 6
Tell One Person

I went back to the house and decided to tell my aunt. I explained to her that I have Hepatitis C, that I can't believe it, and I had to tell somebody. She said, "We will get through this, it's not a death sentence." And I said, "Okay." And she was speaking positive; keeping and trying to keep me positive.

I started to research and research uh all the different things about Hepatitis C. I didn't research anything about cures though because the doctor told me that there was no cure.

All I researched was information about Hepatitis C. I got the statistics and this and that and everything else.

I started changing my eating habits and I was successful with it. It was the main reason I took the tests anyway so I could go to rehab and my mind would be conscious and focused on quitting drinking.

So when I went to the rehab for my drinking problem, it was still on my mind. The rehab center was a very nice place. The people were very friendly. Like I said, it was in the south and the people were very friendly, very nice, very patient.

And as I'm going through this, they asked me if I wanted to check my um my sugar levels, see if I was diabetic. I couldn't understand why they would think that I was diabetic. But they suspected because I was drinking a considerable amount of water not normal for a person that is not diabetic. And I told her, "I don't have diabetes." So she asked me, "Come on, would you like us to check?" So we checked and true enough, I was diabetic.

So, I just found out I had Hepatitis C and found out that I had diabetes soon after. I decided to change all my eating habits to make sure that I address both of them. So as long as I wasn't drinking alcohol, I will be okay. The Hepatitis C, I'll put that on the side and not think about it for a while and I'll concentrate on just the diabetes to get me uh, focused on it.

So I went through rehab. The whole time I was there, I was trying to eat healthier and walk more. When I got out of rehab, I went back to the doctor to get myself checked and to confirm if I have diabetes. And indeed I have; a type two diabetes. I got on pills for my diabetes which wasn't too bad. It was just one pill a day and I could handle that. It wasn't interfering with my Hepatitis C, too.

I explained to the doctors my plan of eating better. I did this for little over a year. As each day went by, I started to think less about hepatitis and only concentrated on the diabetes.

Chapter 7
Life Gets in the Way

I called home back to my reservation in New York, and I found out my mother had cancer. And I decided, "That's it, I am going home, I'm going to take care of my mom." So I went back to New York. After my mom got sick with cancer, all five of us kids moved near her home to help take care of her. For the next year and a half, I took care of my mom.

I was also went to the local health center on the reservation for my medical condition. They explained to me about diabetes, it's treatment and what to expect. They were also giving me my medicine, making sure that I take it. And they had a new doc, uh nurse practitioner, Lori. Lori is super great. She's a great person, she's so thoughtful, nice, uh she kept encouraging me to lose weight, exercise more, and eat healthy. One day she asked me, "Is there um, anything that we might know, might not know about your health, any health issues? Any pains or anything like that?" I said, "No nothing. Oh, I forgot to tell you that I do have Hepatitis C." And she said, "You have what?" I said, "Hepatitis C." At that time, I just accepted what the doctor in Tennessee told me that there was nothing that I could do, that I'll have it, that I shouldn't drink, that there are a couple of things that I couldn't eat and I'll just live with it. And Lori said something that changed my life, "You know, there is a possible cure. There is a treatment for it."

The treatment was twenty six weeks long. I was sitting there thinking, "Treatment? What do you mean treatment?"

So she said that there is a treatment and there's a cure (not guaranteed cure, because there are no guarantees in life) but she said there is a possibility of curing Hepatitis C. And I said, "No, there's no cure." She said, "Yes there is, it's a possibility. But it's twenty six weeks long."

In my next few visits, the nurse practitioner keeps encouraging me to go and meet the doctor and at least get checked and learn some more information. So I made an appointment to see the doctor.

I didn't want to meet the doctor. I did not have any time to spare; I was taking care of my mother full time but I did promise Lori that I will get myself checked. So I ended up going to my appointment. The doctor asked me a few questions and explained more about Hepatitis C. He told me that he would start off by having my old records sent to his office and that I will need to get some blood work done. The doctor also told me that I should attend a class about the treatment. There were a couple of classes offered every week but I decided to go on a Saturday morning. I remember that morning very well. There were only two of us in that room and the other person was really nice. The person conducting the class was explaining what to expect from the treatment, and that it's a twenty six-week long treatment. As I was listening, I started to understand a lot more. The person that was giving the talk explained about side effects, what to expect, and how to deal with each of them. I remember thinking, "I wish I knew someone that had undergone this treatment before so I could ask what it is like." The lady conducting the class told us that she was more worried about the psychological part of the treatment, of how to keep us going for twenty six weeks. Because taking the medicine for twenty six weeks is simple but the psychological effect of the long treatment is the hard part. The psychological effects vary in each person. Some get really sick; others keep on going because stopping means it's less likely that you're going to get cured.

When the class ended, I remember thinking, "There is no

way I can get treatment and take care of my mother at the same time."

I thought to myself, "Well, I'm not going to do this treatment, it's too long and the psychological part just seems to be too much to handle." So I went home to take care of my mother.

But every time I go to the health center, my nurse practitioner kept urging me to get the treatment but I kept putting it off. I did that for a year and a half.

Well, I can say that my family and I took the best care of my mother. We made her as comfortable as we possibly could. She underwent chemo and radiation so I saw what they look like and what they can do to your body. They are cure but also make you sick at the same time. It's hard when somebody you love so much is going through so much pain and there's nothing you can do. My mother was in so much pain. She was so sick and her hair was falling out. The day came where she couldn't take the treatment anymore and she just said, "Okay well there's no more pain of the chemo," and my um, my mother passed away October the tenth at 9:15AM. My mother lost her battle with cancer.

Chapter 8
Treatment and Cure

I didn't want to have relapse on alcohol and drugs, and I know the best way to do it is to stay away from all places or things that may trigger or may cause a moment of weakness. So I went and stayed at a different reservation where I didn't know that many people. It was a lot easier to stay sober when there's nobody around me with alcohol or drugs, and um I stayed there for a few months till I started to feel a little bit better and confident about my sobriety. It was after New Year when I got back.

I went back to my doctor's office to have a check up on my diabetes. She also mentioned that there's a new treatment for Hepatitis C. It's a twelve-week treatment, instead of twenty six. I said, "Well, I can handle twelve weeks." That time I was thinking that it is going to be the same as what my mother went through. So I said, "Well if my mother could handle it, I could handle it as well." So I went ahead and made an appointment. I was told I have to get some blood work done but I kind of put it off again. It was my eldest brother who reminded me about the promise I made to my mother - that I would go and get it done. So I made my appointment again. It was actually a few weeks later but I finally got one. I had my blood work done and the doctor ordered treatment and said that it will be shipped directly to me and that I had to sign when I received it.

I remember the package came in a big, white foam cooler, about one foot by one foot square meter in size so it was not too big. I cut the sides and the tape holding the lid down. I opened it up and there was an envelope in a plastic bag with the instructions in it. I pulled it out and there were some towels below it. I pulled the paper towels out. There were also a couple of ice packs which I pulled out. Inside was another Ziploc bag which contains the pens that are part of the treatment.

So I pulled them out of the bag and put them in the refrigerator right away. Then I pulled the ice packs out and saw two bottles of pills. I then read the instructions. I decided I was going to start my treatment on Saturday night, that way I'll be sick on Sunday and I wouldn't miss time from work and I wouldn't have to see many people.

I had to take the pills twice a day and I set my phone alarm so I will not forget. I did not want to mess this up at all.

I even bought one of those pill cases so I would know if I have taken the dose yet or not. I also kept all the info of all my meds in a box next to my bed and told my friends and family that if anything happens to me, to bring the box with them to the hospital so the doctors would know what I was taking and how much I was taking.

Saturday came and I started taking my pills as directed. Before I gave myself a shot of the pen, I watched a video on YouTube about how to use it just to make sure that I do it right.

I gave myself my first shot and it didn't hurt at all. I honestly didn't even feel it. Then I went to bed.

When I woke up the following morning, I didn't realize that it was exactly six months after my mother passed away. Later that evening, the whole family got together to have a big dinner.

I was sick all day just like what the doctor explained to me.

The doctor said that the effects of the first dose of treatment will be the worst. I was so sick and my bones ached. It felt like my bones were on fire. My mouth tasted disgusting and I was sweating. I also had diarrhea. I couldn't hold anything down, and I had to pretend like everything's okay in front of my family because I didn't tell my family, only my one brother knew about it. And so I spent the whole time faking I was okay but thinking, "Please just go home."

I didn't want to be rude and it was nice to hang out with my family but I was just feeling so sick. I was thinking, "Oh my goodness, I can't believe how sick I got." After the party, everybody left and my brother told me, "Well you need to get up and move around."

I don't think he understood how much pain I was feeling. My bones ached from head to foot. I tried to do some things but it just hurt a lot when I move. I ended up hopping to the shower to see if it would make me feel better. Actually, it did make me feel a little bit better. I couldn't take anything for the pain though because it will not be good for my liver. As soon as I found out that I had Hepatitis C, I stopped taking aspirin, ibuprofen, other pain killers and alcohol. I wouldn't take them for nothing, nothing, nothing. I was very good at it because I was trying to keep my liver running as good as it could possibly can. So I just stayed in bed the rest of the day and tried to sleep the pain off.

The next day, I still couldn't hold anything down. But I felt a lot better though. I continued faking feeling good and did normal things.

I still had that nasty taste in my mouth. I brushed my teeth 10 times every day but the nasty taste won't go away.

I didn't get too much sleep on the 2nd night but it wasn't too bad. And by the third day, I was feeling much, much better that I could eat. By the end of the third day, I didn't even think about being sick. I continued to take my pills as directed and on time every day. I was very good at it. I set my phone alarm at noon and midnight so it is easier to remember. And in cases that I don't have my phone with me, I had a little pill box as back up to make sure that I take the right dose. I wanted to make sure that everything is right. I did this for the first week and when the time for the next pen injection treatment came, I was just by myself again. I didn't want to do it. I didn't want to be sick like that again but I remembered the doctor telling me that it gets easier in the succeeding treatments and that the first one's the hardest. So, I injected it a little bit earlier this time. The next day, it wasn't as bad; it was tolerable. My bones still ached, I was still sweating, and I still got a little bit of diarrhea, but they are not as bad as the first time. I had a real bad taste in my mouth again though and I still couldn't eat. So, I was sick on Sunday, but it was tolerable. When Monday came, it wasn't as bad, and I felt much better come Tuesday; I was back to normal. I said, "Okay, well that's even easier." The third week came and I took my medicine all week long and then came Saturday - time for the pen. I injected it and on the next day, there was no more diarrhea, no more sweats, um and that week I started to eat better. What I would do is I'd eat very bland food like plain rice or plain pasta because I had such a bad metallic taste in my mouth. I still had to brush my teeth ten times a day. I started to learn how to eat. What I meant by that is, instead of eating a whole plate of food, I would eat a quarter of a plate then I'd lie down and wait about fifteen or twenty minutes then eat another quarter of it and then stop. Wait another fifteen or twenty minutes before eating another quarter of it again.

The first two weeks wasn't like that because I didn't know the tricks yet but I learned as I go through it.

I still didn't take any ibuprofen or any pain killer. By the fourth week, I was getting the hang of it and just repeated the same process.

The meds are enough for four weeks only. So I called the number for more meds. It is also a reminder that it's time to go to my doctor and have some blood work done.

I went to my doctor and narrated to him the side effects and everything that I experienced. He asked me how bad the pain was.

I said, "The only way I could describe it is as if you were

in a car on a road trip for five or six hours and you try to get up and your back hurts, all is tight, and it hurts." I said, "You can walk around and you can even fake feeling well but my bones ached a little. I also got a bad taste in my mouth." And that was pretty much the side effects. My hair got a little bit thinner and my nails got so brittle.

When I bumped my pinkie toe, the nail came off. As I was telling him this, he said, "The medicine is doing that." I'm diabetic so I should be very cautious with my feet. I wore boots everywhere I go because I wanted to protect my feet.

My nails hurt a lot, too. Lines grew into the side of my nails, The doctor said, "Why don't you take some ibuprofen?" I told him, "Well, when I found out I have Hepatitis C,

I read about it. I stopped taking aspirin, acetaminophen, ibuprofen, and alcohol because they destroy your liver." I told him I wouldn't take it.

I would rather go through the pain.

He explained to me that everything should just be in moderation. When you're sick like that, you can take a couple of ibuprofen. He told me how much to take. (I am no doctor so ask your doctor if you can take them and how much to take.)

I went home and started the next week of treatment. I took

the pills all week long and then when it was time for the injection, I was ready because everything I needed (like food, water, stuff for brushing my teeth, and protecting my nails) were on my side. It was a lot easier because I could take some ibuprofen for the back pain.

I continued to fake I am doing alright; I didn't tell anybody except for one friend. He would always make sure that I had ibuprofen and that I had stuff to drink, mostly water. He always made sure I had all that.

It got easier and easier as I learned all the little things that I had to do to make life easier and better.

Now, I will tell you this part so you won't stop the treatment.

The fourth week that I got my blood work done, my doctor told me great news that there was no trace of Hepatitis C anymore. He didn't say "cured" but he said no trace. I believe that doctors are not allowed to say cured. He told me we're going to do more check-ups every four weeks which is minimal and helped me along the way. Like I said, it was more important to prepare for the psychological part than the taking of the medicine. The taking of the medicine was easy, I set my phone and made sure I had all that stuff, I made sure there was food ready, and I just kept taking my treatment. So the fifth, sixth, seventh, eighth week went by, and it just got so much easier. After every 4 weeks, I ordered more medicine, and I will get them in the same white, one foot square meter size box and put the contents in the refrigerator right away. Don't mess with that, do it right away. Make sure you talk to your doctor about it. That's uh my treatment and so far so good, all the blood work comes back as negative. There's no trace of Hepatitis C. I tell people I'm cured and like I said, the doctors might not be able to say the word cured but to me, I'm cured.

As far as the side effects, I now have trouble with concentration and memory (I forget things easy).

I feel good and I feel confident. A good side effect was I lost weight - I lost about fifteen pounds. I feel more energetic and much happier. I no longer have depression. There was a point that I was depressed, a side effect of having Hepatitis C as mentioned in the earlier part of the book. But I'm feeling a whole lot better now; a lot more confident and more secure with myself.

I've wanted to write this to explain what I went through and to give hope to others who are experiencing the same disease that I had.If you want me to come and speak in your event, or want to ask me a question, just go to my website: http://DennisClause.com